Anxiety

How a woman can claim back the energy consumed in anxiety and unlease it in a positive way

Melissa Keane – Health Secrets for her

Introduction

I would like to thank you for downloading the book, *"Anxiety"*.

This book has actionable information on how to fight anxiety as a woman.

Women worry; a lot! We are so concerned about literally every aspect of our life and other peoples' lives (even if we know this is none of our business) that we often limit ourselves in so many ways in fear of making a fool of ourselves, not being liked and so much more. We even worry about why we worry so much. We want to make things perfect and rehearse life more often than not. And unless there is no other option, sometimes we would rather stay behind the shadows then celebrate in hidden corners than be the ones on the spotlight just to avoid making one tiny mistake that ruins everything we've spent hours, days, weeks or even months preparing.

Besides, as women, we may often go through lots of good but intrinsically traumatizing experiences in life like giving birth and having cramps. At times, we may be raped or go through other life situations that often increase our fear of uncertainty that we often find ourselves incapable of doing many things that other people do effortlessly. We want to change, but the change is not instant.

We stand before the mirror countless times talking to ourselves (thinking we are addressing a crowd or talking to strangers) but when we are put in situations that put our practice to test, we feel helpless; everything we had practiced goes to the wind. Well, we know that this is unhealthy because if we want to go far in life, we cannot be living a life full of limitations.

That's where this book comes in to walk you through the journey to understanding why you do what you do i.e. have heightened fear of things you know are unreal and how to overcome all that.

Thank you again for downloading this book. I hope you enjoy it!

Best,

Melissa Keane

Table of Contents

An Understanding Of Anxiety

Anxiety can be defined as a state of apprehension or uneasiness. If you suffer from anxiety disorder, you experience a number of symptoms such as excessive worry and fear about issues that shouldn't be a source of worry and fear in the first place. This extreme anxiety always results in severe panic attacks, or a sudden rush of an uncontrollable fear often accompanied by certain physical symptoms such as excessive sweating, a pounding heart, and rapid breathing. Anxiety becomes disabling when it becomes excessive and something to be dreaded every day.

According to Futurity.org, anxiety is so prevalent around the world that 1 in every 13 people has one form of anxiety or another. That is around 7.6% of the world's population, which if we estimate the world's population to be around 7 billion, this translates to over half a billion people suffering from anxiety. To put this into perspective, half a billion is the entire US population plus Mexico and The United Kingdom!

Despite anxiety being treatable, only one-third of people with anxiety get treatment. Unfortunately, if anxiety is not addressed early, people with anxiety disorder are more likely to be hospitalized for mental-related problems. Whether you are suffering from generalized anxiety disorder, panic disorder, obsessive-compulsive disorder (OCD), society anxiety disorder, or posttraumatic disorder, anxiety can affect many other aspects of life like your happiness, satisfaction, and your chances of success in life.

According to several studies, anxiety is more prevalent in women than in men. In fact, if you are a woman, you are twice more likely to suffer from anxiety than a man. This makes it critical to know how to manage anxiety before it gets out of hand. This book looks at the different causes of anxiety including hormonal imbalances and natural ways to treat anxiety.

Anxiety In Women: Why Anxiety Is More Prevalent In Women

According to available statistics, the rate of anxiety among women has been found to be twice the rate in men. The reason behind the high rate of anxiety among women is due to a number of things.

For starters, reproductive events in a woman's life lead to hormonal changes that have been linked to anxiety. For example, the increase in progesterone and estrogen that happens during pregnancy can increase a woman's risk of OCD.

Furthermore, a number of studies indicate that women are more likely to experience mental and physical abuse in their life than men are and abuse has been linked to one developing anxiety disorders.

In addition, men and women handle problems differently. While men actively look for solutions to their problems, women tend to focus so much on their problems and this can make them prone to anxiety disorders. This is mainly because of differences in amygdala activity.

Amygdalae are two almond shape nuclei deeply located within your brain's temporal lobes. Researches have shown that amygdala plays a key role in processing decision-making, memory, and all emotional reactions. Amygdala manages memory storage depending on the intensity of the emotional reactions that accompany the memory. Some studies refer to amygdala as the brain's major processing center for fear.

The amygdala at the right hand side of your brain is responsible for action, which explains why it is most active in men and less active in women while the one on the left hand side is mostly responsible for storing traumatic memories details and inspires more thoughts than action.

The left-hand side amygdala is known to be more active in women and less active in men. This left-hand side amygdala is also known to be more active in anxiety patients. Once triggered, amygdala sends distress messages to all major parts of your brain. Since the worrying part of the human brain is more active in women than in men, it is not surprising that women are more prone to anxiety disorders than men are.

In addition to differences in amygdala increasing the prevalence of anxiety in women, other factors may cause anxiety in women. Let us look at these:

Common Causes Of Anxiety In Women

Most of the causes of anxiety in women are linked to hormones and hormonal interactions and changes that take place during monthly menstrual cycles, pregnancy, and menopause. For instance, estrogen is a common steroid hormone known for its importance in female sexual development and reproduction. It is also known to influence the functions of your brain through its interaction with serotonin, to regulate your mood changes.

Naturally, your body is known to produce more estrogen than a man's body. You are also more likely to experience many changes in your hormonal levels, which may manifest in your sudden mood swings at certain critical periods every month. This regular change in your hormonal levels can cause an imbalance in your serotonin levels, which in turn increases your feelings or fear, anxiety and stress.

Other causes of anxiety include:

Hypothyroidism

Hypothyroidism is a situation that involves the slowing down of your body's cellular metabolism, which reduces the levels of the neurotransmitter known as gamma-aminobutric acid (GABA).

This neurotransmitter has a soothing effect, which is known to prevent the brain from being overly stimulated. Low levels of this neurotransmitter have been linked to mood swings, panic attacks, and anxiety. Some common causes of hypothyroidism include autoimmune diseases like Hashimoto's thyroiditis, medications like lithium, radiation therapy like radiation used to treat cancer of neck and thyroid gland. Common symptoms of the condition include fatigue, dry skin, weight gain, constipation, muscle weakness, heavier than normal menstrual periods, slowed hear rate, thinning hair, muscle aches and increased sensitivity to coldness.

Estrogen Deficiency

Estrogen deficiency occurring simultaneously with menopause can easily lead to anxiety. Estrogen is known to calm the fear response in women, so when your estrogen level is low, your anxiety level becomes heightened.

Excessively High or Low Testosterone

Testosterone is known to be a steroid sex hormone that helps you sustain a healthy libido. When your testosterone level is too high or too low, it increases the secretion of the stress hormone cortisol, which reduces your serotonin levels, increases your amygdala activities thereby increasing your anxiety levels. Some common causes of low testosterone levels include oral contraceptives, age and organ failure.

Low Serotonin Levels

Serotonin is the neurotransmitter with the highest link to anxiety. When your serotonin levels are adequate, you will often feel relaxed, but low serotonin levels have been linked to high anxiety levels in women. Serotonin levels can become low or out of balance following some natural stages that come with hormonal changes in women such as menopause. Imbalance in your level of serotonin can also happen due to your emotions. When your serotonin level is low, your brain tends to produce more of the fear neurotransmitters such as Epinephrine, which increases your anxiety levels.

Low Dopamine Levels

For ages, the role of this neurotransmitter in anxiety in women was not known until recently. Some recent studies suggest that women who have low levels of the feel-good hormone are at a high risk of experiencing anxiety disorders.

Birth Control

There seems to be a correlation between the way your body behaves when you are on certain birth control pills and the way it does when you have low estrogen levels. Certain birth control pills have been found to reduce your estrogen levels and as we mentioned above, low estrogen levels can make you susceptible to developing anxiety disorders.

Other factors

In the last 70 years or thereabout, there have been major shifts in cultural values and thought patterns, which have placed a lot of pressure on women's values and expectations. The society today places so much value on money and status, and you are expected to do whatever it takes to be a perfect wife and mother, make some money to help pay the bills, do most of the chores at home, maintain a great physique, amongst other things. Often, it is hard to live up to these expectations the society and your family places on you. And anxiety is sure to set in due to your inability to meet these expectations as a result of several factors. When you then add up the ever-present gender discrimination and sexism to the above-mentioned factors, anxiety becomes almost unavoidable.

In the following chapters, we are going to look at natural ways to treat anxiety and give you that peace of mind you yearn so bad.

Foods That Can Help Treat Anxiety

Whatever you eat has a huge impact on your general health. Thus, you can eat to manage anxiety and feel good. Here are foods that are known to help with managing anxiety:

Oyster

A number of researches show a correlation between imbalance in the ratio between certain essential minerals such as copper and zinc with anxiety. An increase in copper levels and a decrease in the amount of zinc from your diet could lead to anxiety symptoms. Since oysters are known to be rich in zinc, they can be a good source of this essential mineral to balance the ratio and prevent anxiety.

Full-Fat Kefir

Your gut is believed to be a kind of second brain because it houses over 95% of serotonin. Therefore, the health of your gut is very vital to the effective management of your anxiety symptoms since it contains more than a million neurons. Kefir, high in good bacteria can help keep your brain and gut in good shape to treat anxiety. Kefir also contains important fat-soluble vitamins such as A, B and K2 which are healthy vitamins for the brain.

Chamomile Tea

For a natural calmness when you are dealing with anxiety symptoms, drink some Chamomile tea. This tea has a soothing effect that can help you reduce your anxiety symptoms significantly within a few weeks.

Turmeric

Turmeric contains an antioxidant known as curcuminoids, which is known for its neuroprotective ability that helps improve your mood. It is a very effective option for treating most severe depressive disorders, which has close links with anxiety disorders.

Turkey

You will find this one hard to believe. Have you ever felt calm after eating turkey probably during thanksgiving? That feeling of calmness you get after enjoying turkey comes from the tryptophan. Tryptophan is the natural precursor to the neurotransmitter serotonin known for its ability to help you calm down.

Rooibos Tea

This is a red bush tea mostly found in Africa. It serves as a delicious drink that clams you down. This tea calms you down by balancing your body's major stress hormone, cortisol.

Avocados

Avocados are regarded as super fruits and for good reason; they are not only high in healthy fats but also great at keeping your brain in good health and fighting anxiety. This is due to their high level of B vitamins and certain monounsaturated fats that sustain the health of neurotransmitters and the brain. They also contain an adequate amount of potassium, which reduces high blood pressure naturally.

Dark Chocolate

Over the years, there have been speculations about the health risks people who love chocolates expose themselves to. However, studies have shown that if you take about 1.5 ounces of dark chocolate per day, you will feel much calmer than a person who does not.

Organ Meats

Organ meats are ideal for supplying your body with nutrients such as vitamin D and zinc that can help you fight anxiety. The liver, for instance contains an adequate amount of B vitamins, which are vital for a process known as methylation, a metabolic process in your body which is responsible for the synthesis of the main neurotransmitters that are in charge of regulating your mood.

Foods high in omega-3 fatty acids

Brain health and anxiety are often linked with inflammations. Studies have shown that Omega-3 fats help reduce inflammation. They also help prevent adrenaline and cortisol from spiking. Foods that are rich in Omega-3 include grass-fed beef and fatty fish.

Asparagus

This vegetable is known to be quite rich in sulfur and contains the essential B vitamin known as folic acid. Some cases of neurotransmitter impairments have been linked to low folic acid levels, and this condition can cause anxiety. Asparagus also has moderate amounts of potassium that is essential in reducing high blood pressure.

Leafy Green vegetables

We are constantly told to increase our intake of leafy green vegetables and this is for good reason. Leafy green vegetables are not only high in vitamins and fiber but are also high in minerals like magnesium that helps regulate the adrenal axis of the brain. Adrenal glands are known to produce the stress hormone, cortisol; hence, if they are not well regulated, you increase your risk of anxiety. Some great leafy green vegetables include spinach and Swiss chard.

Meditation Techniques For Treating Anxiety

Most women with anxiety problems may not be willing to try relaxation exercises because they do not believe they can benefit from them. However, it is important to point out that these relaxation exercises can work for anyone, as long as you get yourself adequately prepared for the exercise and have the right attitude towards it. Here are some tips to help you meditate effectively and ease anxiety:

Be committed: Most meditation techniques for anxiety relief take a couple of weeks before you can master them. They are not exercises you could simply try a few times and expect to get instant results. Expecting results so early into meditation will only add to your stress and increase your anxiety. Getting yourself prepared for meditation and knowing that it will take a while before you can experience the results makes you patient and consistent.

Have an open mind and a positive mental attitude: At first, all these meditation techniques might make you feel a little bit silly and awkward, especially if this is your first time attempting them. However, it is important you keep your mind open and believe it is going to be worth every time and effort you put into it in the end.

If you don't believe it can help you, don't start: First convince yourself that this can actually help you get rid of anxiety before your start. Once you doubt the ability of these meditation techniques to help you relax and feel less anxious, then they won't work for you.

Commit at least 20 minutes daily to these meditation techniques. Always ensure you are in a comfortable chair, clothes and under favorable conditions where it is neither too hot nor too cold.

How To Meditate For Stress Relief

Close your eyes: Begin by breathing very calmly. Use your whole diaphragm and breathe in lowly and calmly with your eyes shut. The trick is to first fill your stomach before your chest. Ensure you breathe in and out very slowly. When your lungs are filled with air, hold your breath for some seconds before breathing out. Take in breaths through your nose and let them out through pulsed lips as if you are whistling. You have to practice this breathing technique until you master it before moving on to the subsequent steps.

Count backwards from 5-1: You can count either aloud or in your mind. Whenever you get to one, begin all over again. Don't forget the importance of a controlled, slow measured breathing. You will breathe more slowly if you count slowly. Repeat this counting step until your mind stops concentrating on disturbing thoughts.

Concentrate on Your Body: Try concentrating on how your body feels. Notice which areas of your body seem tensed and focus on them to help them relax. At this point, you will feel your body slumping deeper into the chair you are sitting on and your muscles letting go. This is a feeling of your body going limp as if you have lost your bones.

Turn Off Every Muscle: The only way you can accomplish the previous step is to make sure you turn off your muscles one after the other. You can begin with your right foot. Relax that foot by imagining that it feels weak and heavy. After that, move on to your left foot, and back to your right foot. Alternate between your two feet for a while before moving up until you have reached your face. Repeat the whole process until you feel every muscle turned completely off.

Begin to visualize: Transport yourself to a mentally relaxing spot. Make sure your eyes remain shut all through this process. Imagine yourself in a beautiful park, beach, island, shore, garden, etc. Imagine this beautiful place using all your senses. Pay attention to every detail such as the smell of the flowers, the sunshine, the cool breeze, the humming birds, the color of the water; let this location envelope you completely. Remember to keep on breathing deeply.

Wipe Away Every Negative Thought: Whenever you feel a negative thought creeping into your imagination, imagine the negative thought turning into an object and imagine a relaxing gentle breeze blow it away. A stressful spouse for instance, could be blown away by a gentle breeze until he is out of sight, then go back to imagining the beautiful world surrounding you.

Affirm positively: Begin to give yourself some positive suggestions and affirmations to help distract your mind from negative thoughts and provide you with positive things to think about. This might be the quite awkward but you will be glad you did it. Here are some examples of positive affirmations you could use:

"I'm having a super happy day."

"I'm the best of my kind."

"I feel serene and calm."

"I have a pleasing personality."

"I will get rid of my anxiety completely."

"I'm in love with my life."

"I'm in love with my body."

"I believe in me so much."

Continue your positive affirmations until your negative thoughts fade away.

Yoga And Anxiety: Yoga Poses For Anxiety Relief

Before you can get started on different yoga poses to relieve anxiety, you will need the following yoga props: a small pillow or two yoga blocks, a rolled up towel or bolster, a rolled up hand towel or an eye pillow, and one blanket.

Here are some yoga poses to help you keep your anxiety under control.

The seated Lotus Pose

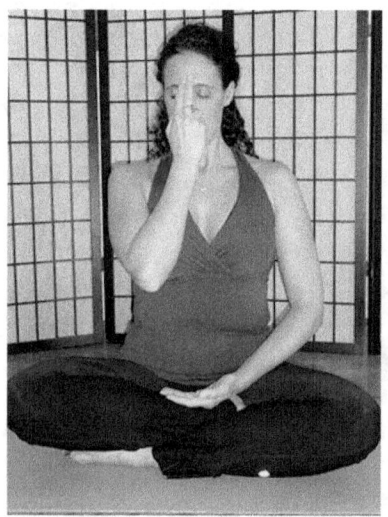

One of the most noticeable signs of anxiety is its effect on your breathing. Whenever you receive any information that should make you anxious or anything that makes you feel threatened, it is common for you to start breathing in faster and shallowly or even hold your breath completely. Assuming this yoga pose and alternating your breathing helps you get a hold of your breathing pattern and makes sure your brain receives adequate supply of oxygen-rich blood.

How to go about this yoga pose

1. Assume a seated position with legs crossed while keeping your spine straight. If you have started feeling the effects of anxiety already, you can ground yourself by resting against a wall with pillows under your knees.

2. Begin by placing your left hand on your lap. Bring the index and middle fingers of the right hand to rest in between your eyebrows. Alternate your breathing by closing the right nostril with your thumb and close the left nostril using the inside of your ring finger. You can hold both nostrils occasionally.

3. Start by taking in deep breaths through your two nostrils and breathing out deeply through both nostrils as well. Then, hold your right nostril and inhale using only your left nostril and count 1-2. Again, hold your two nostrils closed and count 1-6. Then, leave your right nostril while still holding your left nostril and count 1-4. Then breath in through your right nostril and count from 1-2, hold your two nostrils and count from 1-6 and exhale through your left nostril counting 1-4. Repeat the entire process for two minutes.

Legs on the wall pose

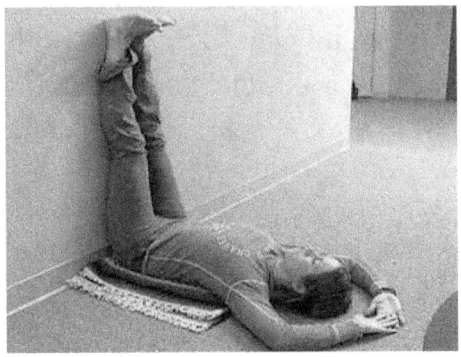

To do this yoga pose effectively, you will need an open wall space, a yoga bolster or a rolled up towel.

1. Sit with the left side against the wall.

2. Bring your body to the left and your legs up on the wall.

3. Lower your bag to the floor, then place your bolster or rolled up towel under your hips at your sacrum region. Make sure your legs are stretched upward completely while your toes face the ceiling. Allow your arms to lie slightly to your side. If you feel anxious, get your palms facing the floor. Place a blanket over you if you feel vulnerable. You can stay in this pose for 5-15 minutes.

The Bridge Pose

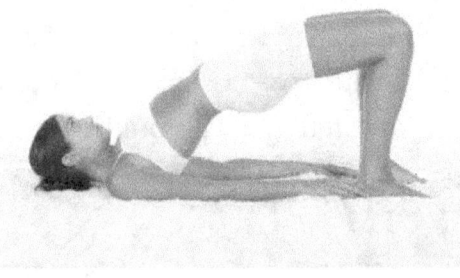

1. Keep your knees in a bent position and place them hip-width apart. Ensure you keep your feet in a parallel position with your arms placed alongside you while facing your palms downwards.

2. Press your palms down, raise up your pelvis, and keep your bottom tightly squeezed.

3. Hold this pose while you take between 5-10 breaths. You can use a yoga block to support your bridge pose until you are able to do this pose without any support. Place the yoga block under your sacrum a little bit above your tailbone. Rest on the block with your lower back.

Maintaining this inverted posture will supply your brain with blood rich in oxygen, which gives your brain a feeling of calmness.

The Child Pose

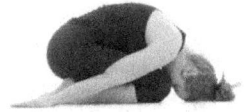

1. Begin the child pose by sitting on your knees.

2. Bring your torso to the mat by bending forward with your arms outstretched. If you feel discomfort in your knees discomfort, try opening them up to make a "V". You can equally wrap your arms alongside you while facing your palms in an upward position. If you are still not comfortable with this pose, place a pillow under your torso to help bring you closer to the floor.

As an alternative, you can assume a puppy pose with your bottom aligned with your knees to create an angle of 90 degrees using your lower legs. You can also drape your lower back using your blanket to keep you grounded and warm.

The Reclining Bound Angle Pose

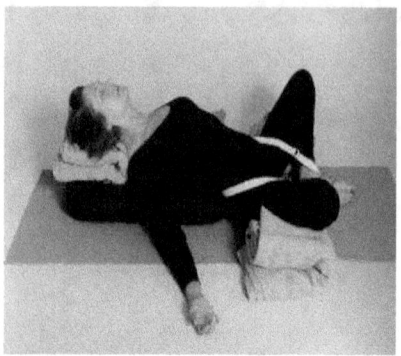

1. Start this pose while in a seated position. Keep a bolster or rolled up blanket at the back of your tailbone.

2. Gently lie down on the bolster or blanket, and keep your feet together while opening your knees in a butterfly pose. If you need knee support, place your yoga pillows or blocks under each one of your knees.

3. You can either place your arms on your stomach or outstretch them to your sides, while allowing your heart and chest to remain open.

In order to benefit from complete relaxation from this pose, you can cover yourself with a blanket and a rolled up hand towel or an eye pillow over your eyes.

The Crocodile Pose

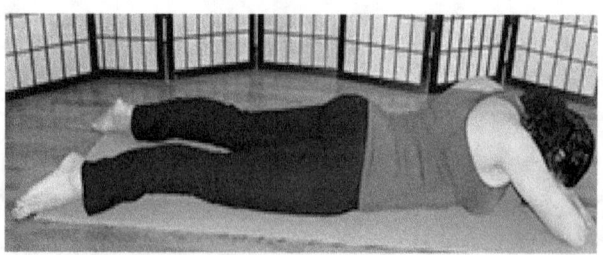

This pose has a deep relaxing effect and helps you breathe deeply from your diaphragm.

1. Start by lying with your face down on your mat.

2. Keep your legs a bit wider than normal hip-distance with your heels pointing inwards and your toes going upwards.

3. Bring your arms and keep them folded in front of you with each hand wrapping around the elbow opposite to it.

4. Now, start drawing your elbows a little closer to you until the upper back is no longer on the floor. Keep your forehead resting on your forearms. Your belly will easily rest on the floor.

5. Start taking in deep breaths from your abdomen. This pose helps your abdomen relax, which enables you to expand into your lower back. In order to release tension from your neck and shoulders, you can place a rolled up towel under your armpits and under your upper chest. You can hold this crocodile pose for around 5-10 minutes.

Half Moon Pose

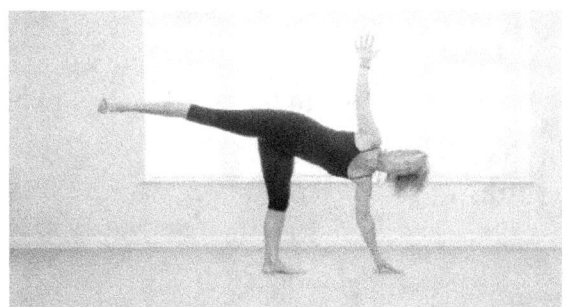

The half moon yoga pose is most ideal for quieting your mind and cultivating focused awareness. The half moon pose is simply a balancing posture that requires you to raise one of your legs, preferably the right leg at about 90 degrees with one of your hands and the other leg on the floor or on a block and one hand raised as high as it can go. This type of balancing yoga pose helps shift your attention from your mind to your body.

Supported Shoulder Stand

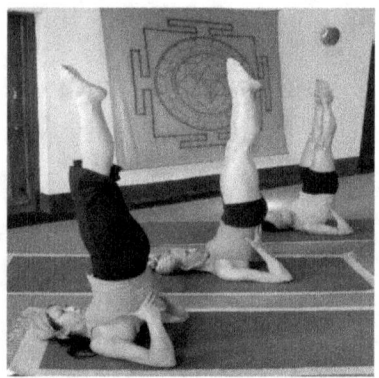

This yoga pose works on the principle of inversions. When you stand on your head or your shoulder, it helps invade your mind and turn everything upside down. Since anxiety mostly works on your perceptions, the feelings of fear and unease you feel will naturally begin to ebb whenever you assume this upside down posture.

Simply lie on your back, raise your two legs up with your two hands supporting your weight at the waist or your lower back. This pose is all about getting out of your mind.

Standing Forward Bend

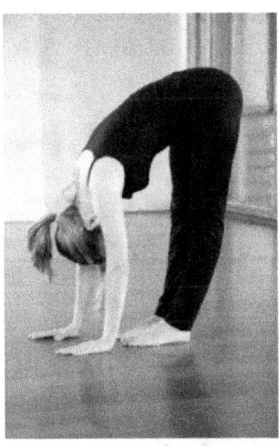

The forward bend yoga pose might look so simple, but it has been found to be a very essential yoga pose for calming your nervous system, which makes it ideal for treating anxiety-related issues. You can either practice it as a lone yoga pose or in-between different yoga poses.

Simply bend down, place your two palms on the floor, with your head in-between your hands, and concentrate on your breathing for a few minutes. You can repeat this occasionally.

Fish Pose

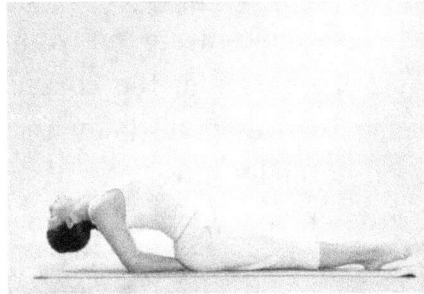

The fish yoga pose is ideal for fighting anxiety and fatigue. As a beginner, it may help to get your thickly folded blanket and place it beneath your head to give support to your neck region.

1. Sit on your mat with your two legs stretched in front of you, and then fall back gradually with your elbows on the floor as a kind of balance.

2. Let your head hang a little bit above the floor while you face upwards. Maintain this pose for about 2 minutes for a start, and then increase it to 3-4 minutes as you become more accustomed to it.

The Corpse Pose

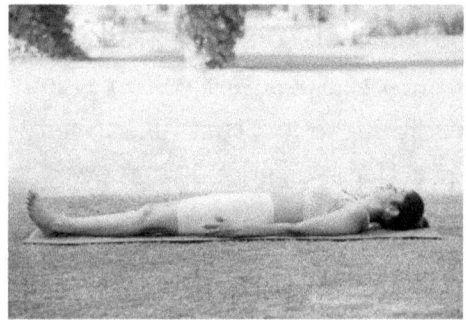

This particular yoga pose is most suitable for the end of your yoga exercises.

Simply lie down on your back when you feel exhausted, with your arms placed at your sides, and concentrate on your breath for 1-10 minutes. In terms of relaxation, the corpse pose remains the ultimate because it gives your body the chance to sink into the ground. Additionally, this yoga pose makes it easier for you to concentrate on your breath by lying still on your back and watching your belly rise and fall in a rhythmic motion.

Make sure you practice these anti-anxiety yoga poses daily to help you relax and manage anxiety. Engaging in some of these exercises will also help you maintain a healthy body and mind, which keeps anxiety away altogether.

Other Natural Remedies For Anxiety

Here are some natural ways to calm yourself when you feel you have an anxiety attack or when you are just too anxious.

Practice Calm Deep Breathing

Abdominal breathing can help relieve you of anxiety. You can engage in deep abdominal breathing for about 20-30 minutes per day to help you regain your lost feeling of calmness. Deep breathing is said to help increase oxygen supply to your brain, and help stimulate your parasympathetic nervous system, which is known to help promote calmness.

Calm breathing requires taking some very smooth regular breaths at a slow pace. Sit upright and breathe in slowly through your nose. Then hold your breath for 1-2 seconds and slowly exhale through your mouth.

Get a Good Massage

Whenever you find yourself feeling unusually anxious, you can ask one of your close friends or your partner to massage your shoulders. Getting a couple of minutes' massage will help get rid of anxiety and stress.

Chew Gum

According to an International Congress of Behavioral Medicine, chewing gum can provide good relief from anxiety, improve mental alertness and relieve stress.

Visit an Art Gallery

One big aspect of treating anxiety and depression is what is known as art therapy. According to studies, looking at beautiful artworks can go a long way to reduce your anxiety levels. Therefore, the next time you feel like you are just too anxious, why not visit the nearest art gallery. Just looking at beautiful works of art will help you remember the beauty of life.

Schedule relaxation time

Find at least 30 minutes to engage in any activity you find relaxing such as walking in the park or some forest reserve where its quiet with birds chirping. You could walk your dog, take your toddler along, walk with your partner, or engage in whatever else you find relaxing.

Use lavender essential oil

According to one study on women who were anxious about a medical procedure they were about to have, researchers found that the number of such women who inhaled some lavender about half an hour before the medical procedure began were much calmer than those who did not.

Thus, to calm yourself, try lavender essential oil. You can either rub it into your temple or put some drops of it on your collarbone. The smell of lavender wafts up and the odor gives you a very relaxing feeling.

It is important you check with your doctor first before using the essential oil.

Keep yourself grounded

According to a marriage counselor and women therapist in Los Angeles, make sure you engage in a tangible activity whenever you experience those panic attacks.

You can take out your house keys and run your fingers along the keys to get a sensation that could give you a "grounding" feeling. Alternatively, you could pick up a paperweight weight and hold it in your hands for a couple of minutes or get an ice cube and hold it for as long as you can endure the freezing sensation.

So how does this work? According to experts, it is not possible for your brain to be in two places at the same time. Any of these activities would keep you distracted from any anxious feelings. Your mind would be shifted from those racing, catastrophic thoughts that go hand-in-hand with anxiety to that cold ice cube in your hand, the paperweight, or the sensation running your fingers along your house keys gives you.

Engage in physical exercises

Certain physical exercises have been found to be quite beneficial as anti-anxiety workouts. Such exercises include aerobic exercises that increase your heart rate. Here are a number of aerobic exercises that can help you control your anxiety levels.

Biking

Brisk walking

Dancing

Tennis

Running

Swimming

Jogging

Conclusion

Thank you again for downloading this book!

I hope this book has helped you understand anxiety better and why as a woman you are more prone to anxiety disorders.

The next step is to try out the different natural techniques for managing anxiety and use what works best for you.

Finally, if you enjoyed this book, would you be kind enough to leave a review for this book on Amazon?

Thank you and good luck!

Best,

Melissa Keane

www.ingramcontent.com/pod-product-compliance
Lightning Source LLC
Chambersburg PA
CBHW061933280526
45787CB00004B/1588